HEALTHY CHRISTIAN LIVING: WEIGH DOWN LIFESTYLE

30 Day Devotional

RUTH VERBREE

KAYCE BROENING

Reeverb Publishing

ISBN: 9781989100172

Preface

Dear Woman Chosen For Greatness,

To get the most out of this devotional, we recommend that in addition to reading one devotional per day, you also spend some time in prayer and reflection and write down your thoughts.

This 30 day devotional is made exactly for where you are at in your journey.

We love you and are praying for you.

Your Sisters and Brothers in Christ,

Weigh Down Lifestyle Team

Day 1

"Do not conform to the pattern of this world, but be transformed by the renewing of your mind. Then you will be able to test and approve what God's will is—his good, pleasing and perfect will."

(Romans 12:2, NIV)

Put Your Oxygen Mask On First

"If the cabin loses pressure, an oxygen mask will drop down from the overhead area. Please put your own mask over your mouth and nose before you try to assist others."

If you have ever flown on a commercial flight, you have heard this phrase before. It is repeated every time the plane takes off without fail. It is a known fact that you are not able to assist anyone else if you cannot breathe yourself.

On your weight loss journey, it is so important to place your oxygen mask on your own face first. I am talking about self-care, the importance of taking care of your own mind, body and soul with all your strength. The Bible speaks to renewing your mind as the first step.

Consider Romans 12:2: "Do not conform to the pattern of this world, but be transformed by the renewing of your mind. Then you will be able to test and approve what God's will is—his good, pleasing and perfect will" (NIV).

First of all, what is a pattern? According to Google, "a pattern is an order or design or prototype."

Our world has many patterns that we live in and learn from. For example, there are mathematical patterns, scientific patterns, creative sewing and art patterns, and language and communication patterns. Wow…we live in a complex patterned world. There are natural God-made patterns too that shape the way we live our lives, like rising in the morning and lying down in the evening. Like the tides of the sea rolling in and rolling out, many things we have no control over.

So what does it mean to not conform to the patterns of this world? Our world has so many patterns that shift our focus away from God and lead us down a life of despair. These patterns are easy to fall into and difficult to escape once we become enslaved in the patterns. Some of these patterns are routines and behaviors that lead us away from the Father. This may be a pattern of neglecting to read the Word, a pattern of turning to alcohol or food for comfort rather than to God. It could mean a pattern of neglecting to care for ourselves; a pattern of forgetting to put on our own "oxygen mask."

When I was spiralling down into depression when caring for my sick husband, I realized that I was forgetting to care for myself. I needed to put my own oxygen mask on so that I was healthy, and then I could also help my hubby. When I started working on loving myself and renewing my mind, I was able to transform my life and focus on other things in my life as well, like putting the right nutrients and the right thoughts into my mind and body. Changing our patterns can completely transform our lives and renew our mind in a positive way.

Renewing your mind can be done in many ways, as in listening to wise teaching, meditating on scripture or maybe enjoying inspirational songs. Positive words and influences are always a key to our success.

Working towards your ideal weight is just another way of putting on your own oxygen mask first. It's important to treat your body well and give it the nutrients it needs so that you have the energy you need to live a happy and healthy lifestyle. It is most certainly a part of God's good, pleasing and perfect will.

Extra Reading

"Do you not know that your bodies are temples of the Holy Spirit, who is in you, whom you have received from God? You are not your own; you were bought at a price. Therefore, honor God with your bodies."

(1 Corinthians 6:19-20, NIV)

Prayer Journal

Take some time to reflect on what this means to you. Write your thoughts in your prayer journal.

Day 2

"For you created my inmost being; you knit me together in my mother's womb. I praise you because I am fearfully and wonderfully made; your works are wonderful, I know that full well."

(Psalm 139:13, NIV)

Your Exquisite Uniqueness

Who hasn't been a little discouraged at some point in their life with the way they look?

I know I have had doubts and been discouraged at times about the way I look. I have had negative thoughts and feelings and different struggles at times in my life. Somehow our culture wants us to believe that we should never grow old, that we must all have the body of a 20-year-old supermodel, wear a size zero, have the six-pack abs, and the dreaded scale should not go above a certain number! The information the world is feeding us is just not true. What is true then?

Firstly, God knows you intimately! Psalm 139:13: "For you (God) created my inmost being, you knit me together in my mother's womb. I praise you because I am fearfully and wonderfully made" (NIV).

Secondly, God knew you before you were born. Psalm 139:16: "Your eyes saw my unformed body; all the days ordained for me were written in your book before one of them came to be" (NIV).

It's important to recognize that God made you who you are, infinitely valuable, and all the exquisite, unique gifts you possess are from him. You should never doubt this. Your character, your innermost thoughts, your spirit, along with your gifts and your talents, make up the unique person you are, including every wrinkle or gray hair on your head. There is not another person on the planet exactly the same as you, not anywhere in the entire universe. That is exciting and profound.

God also wants us to be the healthiest version of who he made us to be. The bible speaks about treating our bodies like a temple and that means taking care of our health too. We don't need to be a supermodel or have abs of steel, but we do need to treat our bodies with love and respect and thank God for making us unique and special.

God loves you for who you are right now and so it's important to love who God created you to be too. Begin to love yourself anew, to treat your body well, and to thank God for making you so exquisitely unique. Without your individuality, you would not be able to carry out the purpose God has planned specifically for you, whatever stage of life you are in.

Extra Reading

"'For I know the plans I have for you," declares the Lord, "plans to prosper you and not to harm you, plans to give you hope and a future."'

(Jeremiah 29:11, NIV)

Prayer Journal

Take some time to reflect on what this means to you. Write your thoughts in your prayer journal.

Day 3

"Who shall separate us from the love of Christ? Shall trouble or hardship or persecution or famine or nakedness or danger or sword?"

(Romans 8:35, NIV)

Think Of A Past Memory

Isn't the gift of memory so great? I often marvel at how God has made us.

Your memories work both ways; your memory can forget some of the bad things or bad times you have experienced, and your memory can remember those pleasant, more fulfilling times, but our memories can definitely sharpen us.

Think of a time when you were in a peaceful setting, maybe you were on vacation soaking up the sun rays on a beautiful beach, maybe you were skiing down a majestic mountain, maybe you were hiking in the woods where you grew up, or maybe you were spending time with family or friends. Doesn't that bring a smile to your face? I know it does for me.

Sometimes simply looking at a picture or the smell of freshly baked bread can be the stimulus to bring back a memory. Maybe it's the sounds you hear in the background or even the touch of an object that can trigger a memory.

As you continue on your weight loss journey, remember the time you first learned about God's deep love for you. This is a memory that can sharpen you. Remember that God wants the best for you. Remember that you are deeply loved by God and there isn't one thing you can do to remove his love for you. Romans 8:35: "Who shall separate us from the love of Christ? Shall trouble or hardship or persecution or famine or nakedness or danger or sword?" (NIV). What a great memory this is!

⸺

Extra Reading

"But because of his great love for us, God, who is rich in mercy, made us alive with Christ even when we were dead in transgressions—it is by grace you have been saved."

(Ephesians 2:4, NIV).

⸺

Prayer Journal

Take some time to reflect on what this means to you. Write your thoughts in your prayer journal.

Day 4

"Do you not know that in a race all the runners run, but only one gets the prize? Run in such a way as to get the prize. Everyone who competes in the games goes into strict training."

(1 Corinthians 9:24-25, NIV)

In Training

If you want to be successful in any part of your life, discipline, motivation and self control are pieces of the puzzle you will need to figure out.

On your weight loss journey, it is important not to use the word "try." Instead of trying to lose weight, think of your journey as being in-training to lose weight. Training has its ups and downs, training has successes and failures, but that is the nature of being in training for something. Athletes have good days and bad days, but they never quit. When you use the word try, you may have the tendency to want to give up, and when you are in-training…you just don't quit!

When we are in-training for life, we are continually working at improving our own journey.

Have you heard that weight loss takes more than willpower? If you put all your energy into willpower, most likely you will fail in a very short time. Think about that donut on the counter in front of you. You can walk past it multiple times, but eventually you decide to take the first bite. It's a slippery slope.

Willpower only lasts for a short time and eventually it wanes, so it's much better to say that you are in-training. If you mess up, you just get up again and train some more. Your training may tell you to place that donut out of sight, so that out of sight is out of mind for the next time. Training works because we learn from our mistakes.

The apostle Paul said in 1 Corinthians 9:24-25: "Do you not know that in a race all the runners run, but only one gets the prize? Run in such a way as to get the prize. Everyone who competes in the games goes into strict training" (NIV).

We need to work towards our goal every day like an athlete who is in training.

As you consider this today, think of the difference between saying to yourself: "I am trying" versus "I am in-training."

These thoughts are very different aren't they? "I am trying" somehow expects defeat, whereas "I am in-train-ing" speaks of improving and moving forward every day. This can make a powerful impact in your journey today.

Extra Reading

"Commit to the LORD whatever you do, and he will establish your plans."

(Proverbs 16:3, NIV)

Prayer Journal

Take some time to reflect on what this means to you. Write your thoughts in your prayer journal.

Day 5

"Surely everyone goes around like a mere phantom; in vain they rush about, heaping up wealth without knowing whose it will finally be."

(Psalm 39:6, NIV)

Take 2

Rush. Rush. Rush! The tyranny of the urgent is what seems to run our lives sometimes. This has been one of the things in our culture which has caused us excess stress, and for many of us has been the cause of extra weight gain. Why? The answer is simple. Rushing causes us to look for the simplest, easiest way to survive. It means fast food solutions where we go through the drive-thru and eat on the run, or we pick up a packaged, convenient meal that we can quickly throw in the oven at home after a long day at work. It's these processed foods with very little nutrition that causes us to crave more. We still feel hungry soon after inhaling the food so we eat more than we need or we eat again soon after our meal. It doesn't take long before we notice our weight creeping up.

Rushing isn't a new thing. King David speaks about the problem of rushing in Psalm 39:6: "Surely everyone goes around like a mere phantom; in vain they rush about, heaping up wealth without knowing whose it will finally be" (NIV).

This describes our world today, don't you think?

What is the solution then? The solution is to take 2 minutes with God when things are spinning out of control. Take yourself to a quiet place. Stand still, or just sit in a chair. Close your eyes and say: "I belong to Jesus. Please give me peace, and help me to make wise choices."

Asking Him to give you the peace that surpasses all under-standing can help you make a wise choice, and in this case it would be a wise food choice. These 2 minutes with God may help you to become more aware of your situation and to become more mindful of what you eat or put in your mouth. It may help you make better choices and will help you not to mindlessly overindulge. It will bring your focus back so that your choices align with your goals.

Learning the ability to take 2 can be a life-changer in many aspects of your life. How will this technique affect your life today?

Extra Reading

"See what great love the Father has lavished on us, that we should be called children of God! And that is what we are!"

(1 John 3:1, NIV)

Prayer Journal

Take some time to reflect on what this means to you. Write your thoughts in your prayer journal.

Day 6

"We are fearfully and wonderfully made."

(Psalm 139:14, NIV)

Your Body Is A Temple

You are a gift from God. If you have had a child, you understand the love for a child. Your child was a gift from God just like you were a gift from God to your parents.

Throughout the many seasons of life, our physical appearance will change, but we can decide today how we take care of our bodies. It's never too late to change that.

Do you look to the scale to tell you what your worth is? Most of us have been guilty of this at one point. Do not let the scale define who you are. "We are fearfully and wonderfully made" it says in Psalms 139:14 (NIV). It's important to look after our bodies. We can rest in peace knowing that God's forgiveness covers all our sins, including the neglect of ourselves.

"Do you not know that your bodies are temples of the Holy Spirit, who is in you, whom you have received from God? You are not your own" (1 Corinthians 6:19, NIV).

This teaches us the importance of having our bodies set apart as an act of worship to God. We can choose to take care of our bodies, not only for longevity, but to remain energized to live out the purpose that God has envisioned for us.

We all have things we would like to change about our bodies, but God loves and cares for us today, just as we are now. He doesn't wait for us to have the perfect body; He loves us unconditionally. You are Enough! God loves you, and God knows that you are creating a healthy life for yourself even now. Eating clean, changing some of your old habits, and learning to love your body is a way of honoring the temple.

Begin to honor your body today as you eat clean, move daily, renew your mind, and grow in the knowledge of His will.

Extra Reading

"So, whether you eat or drink or whatever you do, do it all for the glory of God."

(1 Corinthians 10:31, NIV)

Prayer Journal

Take some time to reflect on what this means to you. Write
your thoughts in your prayer journal.

Day 7

"For we are God's handiwork, created in Christ Jesus to do good works, which God prepared in advance for us to do."

(Ephesians 2:10, NIV)

Self-Love

Self-love has two very different perspectives. Some people think self-love is egotistical and vain, only thinking of yourself, while the other perspective is about self-love being a necessity. Self-love is a necessity in knowing that you need to take care of yourself so that you can better serve those around you and your loved ones, and to do what you were called to do.

I believe that self-love is not selfish at all. It is not vain or conceited, but it is doing what God calls us to do, to take care of our bodies because our bodies are the temple of the Holy Spirit. Self-love is not a moral flaw, not vanity, but is what God desires and intends for us to do, to take care of ourselves.

In order to love your neighbour, you must love yourself first. Self-love actually allows you to make healthy choices. Self-love allows you to take time to move daily. Self-love allows you to read these devotions. Self-love is what allows you to reach your target weight loss goal.

Love yourself today and everyday moving forward.

See how different you feel when you give yourself permission to actually love yourself! You'll be amazed at the difference when you make yourself a priority. Make healthy choices and give yourself some praise. God loves you and loved you so much that He sent His only Son for you. So, it's okay to start loving yourself as well. We can love, because He first loved us.

Extra Reading

"For by the grace given me I say to every one of you: Do not think of yourself more highly than you ought, but rather think of yourself with sober judgment, in accordance with the faith God has distributed to each of you."

(Romans 12:3, NIV)

Prayer Journal

Take some time to reflect on what this means to you. Write your thoughts in your prayer journal.

Day 8

"For in him all things were created: things in heaven and on earth, visible and invisible, whether thrones or powers or rulers or authorities; all things have been created through him and for him"

(Colossians 1:16, NIV)

What Is My Purpose?

What is your purpose? This is a question I'm sure you have struggled with at some point in your life. I know I have. I still find myself asking God this question at times. Jesus told us that His sole purpose on earth was to do the work of his Father. This is what our purpose is also.

What is your purpose? If you believe the Bible, then it is also your purpose to do the will of the Father. So, you might ask, "Father...What is it that you want me to do?"

It is often difficult to fully understand what our purpose is, but it is important to step out in faith knowing that God wants us to act in accordance with His will. Taking action, stepping out in faith requires courage. It's being WILLING to be WILLING.

When you take the leap of faith about your purpose, you jump! It's like jumping off a diving board and trusting that the pool is filled with water. You take that leap of faith. God knows if you are taking action, and He can certainly stop you or turn you around if it is not the right direction. What matters is that we are doing the will of the Father.

Have you lost your purpose? If so, it's time to find it again. When I finally figured out that my purpose was to help women learn to love themselves again and to see that their identity was in Christ and not on a number on the scale, I then began to feel fulfilled and passionate about life again.

What is holding you back? Do you know what your purpose is? If not, I challenge you to ask God what it is He wants you to do with your life? It's certainly NOT over. Your purpose may change through different seasons in life, but you definitely are here for a purpose.

Extra Reading

"Many are the plans in a person's heart, but it is the LORD's purpose that prevails."

(Proverbs 19:21, NIV)

Prayer Journal

Take some time to reflect on what this means to you. Write your thoughts in your prayer journal.

Day 9

"A gentle answer turns away wrath, but a harsh word stirs up anger. The tongue of the wise commends knowledge, but the mouth of a fool gushes folly."

(Proverbs 15:1, NIV)

Difficult People

Do you have any difficult people in your life? In this broken world, difficult people are everywhere. Coworkers or friends are willing to do anything to get ahead. You may have friends who want to sabotage your new lifestyle. You may have family members who are critical of your new food choices or your newfound lifestyle success, or they may be critical of your weight loss or your positive attitude toward life.

Difficult people remind me of the story of Moses in the Bible. He was no stranger to difficult people. He was leading a group of people out of slavery, showing them many miracles and leading them safely away from the

Egyptians, but they were not happy with him. Instead of being grateful for their new freedom and provision from God, they were complaining about the food, grumbling about not having water, wishing they had died in Egypt, and wishing they could choose another leader. Even Moses' own siblings were difficult and complained to God about their brother.

Moses didn't retaliate and defend himself against the harsh accusations. He repeatedly interceded for them. By God's grace he persevered. At the end of his life, he was still lovingly leading these difficult people.

So, what do we do with difficult people in our lives?

Here are some Biblical tips:

- Ask God to soften your heart towards the difficult person in your life. Put up your shield to stop the anger and the desire to want to get even.
- Seek to be kind and to understand that this person may be facing their own struggles and meet them with renewed compassion.
- Pray for the difficult people in your life and ask God to be at work in their hearts.
- Do not be derailed by the difficult people who don't want you to succeed in your plan.
- Set boundaries for yourself and put up your shield against the difficult people in your life.
- Know that with God in your journey, you can succeed!

Extra Reading

"But I tell you, love your enemies and pray for those who persecute you."

(Matthew 5:44, NIV)

Prayer Journal

Take some time to reflect on what this means to you. Write your thoughts in your prayer journal.

Day 10

"Weeping may stay for the night, but rejoicing comes in the morning."

(Psalm 30:5, NIV)

Laughter Is A Medicine

When was the last time you had a good deep belly laugh?

I hope you can recall a laughing spell that took place quite recently. I believe that laughter truly is a medicine that heals the soul.

I recall a time recently when my husband and I spent a weekend together at our friends' house. One evening my friend and I were watching a movie and my girlfriend went to get up out of her lounge chair and she fell down. We both roared with laughter. This does not sound particularly funny as I write this, but I find myself smiling again, because we laughed so hard that we cried. We experienced a true deep belly laugh. What a great memory!

Great memories are wonderful, but a deep belly laugh actually has more benefits to your body than you might realize. Laughter really is like a medicine to the soul. The world-renowned motivational speaker, Les Brown, lives for laughter and says it has been the medicine that has helped him remain healthy throughout his life, even while living with cancer for the last 27 years. The Bible also speaks to this. Proverbs 17:22: "A merry heart does good, like medicine, but a broken spirit dries the bones" (NIV).

God knows about laughter and wants us to experience this pleasure. Scientifically, laughter triggers the release of endorphins and is the body's natural hormone booster. It literally boosts our mood.

There are other benefits as well. Laughter decreases the stress hormones and also boosts your immune system. Laughter burns calories which is a real bonus on our weight loss journey!! Just think…, God created laughter, and He created all the added benefits for your body.

Let's begin to incorporate more laughter into our lives, as this is part of living a happy, healthy life with God at the center. Maybe you need to watch a funny video or read a funny story or get a joke book. It's time to get creative in learning how to laugh again. Humor is one medicine that God prescribes for us in unlimited dosages. Humor yourself today.

The Bible itself has some humor for us to read.

Extra Reading

"Sarah said, "God has brought me laughter, and everyone who hears about this will laugh with me." And she added, "Who would have said to Abraham that Sarah would nurse children? Yet I have borne him a son in his old age."

(Genesis 21:6-7, NIV)

Prayer Journal

Take some time to reflect on what this means to you. Write your thoughts in your prayer journal.

Day 11

"The Lord directs the steps of the godly. He delights in every detail of their lives. Though they stumble, they will never fall, for the Lord holds them by the hand."

(Psalm 37:23-24, NIV)

Falling Forward

Do you remember what dominos are? As a child, I would set them up and watch as they would begin to fall and keep falling forwards. I love the analogy of dominos and how I can relate that to my own life. Dominos falling forward just keep moving forward - they don't quit.

When you are falling forwards, it is a really great thing! Falling forwards is not failure; it is going forwards regardless of whether you have had a few slip ups. I love what Les Brown says, "when you fall down and you can still look up...you can still get up!" Two steps forward and one step back is still one step ahead.

Regardless of whether you have had trials, slip ups, or feel like you're slipping, remember to look up, and then get right back up. Be like the game of dominos and keep falling forwards. Psalm 37:23-24 "The Lord directs the steps of the godly. He delights in every detail of their lives. Though they stumble, they will never fall, for the Lord holds them by the hand" (NIV).

Remember you are not alone on this journey. You have God leading and directing you forward, and with God in the journey it is possible! Together with God's guidance and His loving hand on you, you will get to your target goal each and every day. You can do all things through Christs who strengthens you.

Extra Reading

"They will never hunger or thirst, nor will the desert heat or the sun beat down on them."

(Isaiah 49:10, NIV)

Prayer Journal

Take some time to reflect on what this means to you. Write your thoughts in your prayer journal.

Day 12

"You are the light of the world. A town built on a hill cannot be hidden. Neither do people light a lamp and put it under a bowl. Instead they put it on its stand, and it gives light to everyone in the house."

(Matthew 5:14-15, NIV)

Be The Light

What does it mean to be the light? In Matthew 5:14-16, Jesus compares his followers to light, saying we are "the light of the world," unable to be hidden. No one puts a lamp under a bowl because a lamp is designed to help people see in dark places. Christ followers are like the lamp - we should give light to those around us through our words and actions.

By growing in relationship with Jesus every day, following Him step by step, we partner with Him in spreading the truth and light. Darkness can be defined as the absence of light. Light dispels the darkness and it enables you to see.

God is light, and since He sent His Holy Spirit to live inside of us, we are the light of the world. We dispel the darkness that is around us. As His ambassadors on earth, we shine even when we don't know it. This is really something to ponder. I love the fact that we are the light.

It is my passion to help you grow in your new lifestyle journey to shine brightly. You already have all the gifts you need; God made you in His image. A friend of mine says it this way - You are a creative and compassionate spiritual being currently living in this physical form. You are infinitely valuable, exquisitely unique and perfect in your personhood.

I love helping women succeed in their weight loss journey. I want you to live a happy, healthy life and to be the Light, to be the person God designed you to be. Don't hide your light under a rock. You have so much light to give. The truth of Scripture is that God knows we have imperfections. He knows that we have flaws, that we make mistakes, and we don't need to figure everything out before we can shine our light. It is very freeing to know that God uses us if we are willing to shine our light even though we aren't perfect.

When we live with the courage to be truly vulnerable and honest, we open our lives for all to see the light of God within us. Where you are today does not define where you will be in a month, 6 months, or in a year. Each day we can shine brighter.

Jesus told His followers to "let your light shine before others," calling them to live an active faith, not a passive one. Put your light on its stand. Your circumstances are an opportunity to shine brightly for the Lord and to share God's overcoming truth with those around you. Your family and community can tell what you believe by your everyday actions and in how you live.

Let's shine our lights together.

———

Extra Reading

"In the same way, let your light shine before others, that they may see your good deeds and glorify your Father in heaven."

(Matthew 5:16 , NIV)

———

Prayer Journal

Take some time to reflect on what this means to you. Write your thoughts in your prayer journal.

Day 13

"Be strong and courageous. Do not be afraid or terrified because of them, for the Lord your God goes with you; he will never leave you or forsake you."

(Deuteronomy 31:6, NIV)

Be Strong And Courageous

We all have challenges in our lives. Some of them come from outside sources and some are internal challenges. What challenges are you facing today?

I hope that you will take today's verse and cling to it throughout the day. In 1952, Florence Chadwick attempted to swim the 26 miles between Catalina Island and the California coastline. This was an internal challenge for her. After about 15 hours, a thick fog set in. Florence began to doubt her ability and she told her mother, who was in one of the boats, that she did not think she could make it. She swam for another hour before asking to be pulled out, unable to see the coastline due to the fog. As she sat in the boat, she found out she had stopped swimming just one mile away from her destination. How heart wrenching this must have been for her to realize that her doubt kept her from her goal! Isn't it true that many of us quit on the brink of success?

It is often near the end that we get into that fog which zaps our strength and blurs our focus. Like Florence, sometimes we just give up too soon. This is when we need to keep the pressure on to finish the race, to succeed in the challenge set out before us.

One story in the Bible is where Joshua also faced discouragement and loss of focus. Here are the words he heard from God to keep him going: "Be strong and courageous. Do not be afraid; do not be discouraged, for the Lord your God will be with you wherever you go." (Joshua 1:9, NIV). Wow! What a beautiful promise from the Lord. He will be with you wherever you go.

My goal is to help you to be strong and courageous, to keep you from doubting yourself, to keep you away from the fear of failure, and to encourage you each step of the way every day. I know that you have probably doubted yourself or doubted decisions that you have made in the past just like Florence. You have doubted that you could get up again after being knocked down. You may have doubted that you could lose weight. You have doubted that you could win the race set out before you.

The encouraging words from the bible tell us to let go and let God guide us. When we allow God to guide us and we keep our focus on Him, the doubt vanishes. We need to be strong and courageous and we will reach our goals. The Lord is with us today wherever we go, just like He was with Joshua!

Extra Reading

"Be strong and very courageous. Be careful to obey all the law my servant Moses gave you; do not turn from it to the right or to the left, that you may be successful wherever you go. Keep this Book of the Law always on your lips; meditate on it day and night, so that you may be careful to do everything written in it. Then you will be prosperous and successful. Have I not commanded you? Be strong and courageous. Do not be afraid; do not be discouraged, for the Lord your God will be with you wherever you go."

(Joshua 1:7-9, NIV)

Prayer Journal

Take some time to reflect on what this means to you. Write your thoughts in your prayer journal.

Day 14

_____

"My thoughts are not your thoughts, neither are your ways my ways."

(Isaiah 55:8, NIV)

God Answers Prayer

Prayer changes things. Maybe you've heard that statement before but the question is…do you believe it?

You may have heard ministers preach on today's verse: "The prayer of a righteous person is powerful and effective" (James 5:16, NIV). Maybe you've heard testimonies of people who said the power of prayer affected their own lives or the lives of others. And… maybe you want to believe what the Bible teaches about prayer. Sometimes that's difficult.

Have there been times when you prayed and nothing seemed to happen? Why would God answer one person's prayer while apparently ignoring the prayer of someone else? There is no human answer to such questions. But one thing we do know is that God hears each one of our prayers when we call on him. AND we know God answers our prayers. Maybe it's not always the answer we want, but our God is a listening God and He answers in His own way, according to His plans. As God reveals through the prophet Isaiah: "My thoughts are not your thoughts, neither are your ways my ways" (Isaiah 55:8, NIV).

I understand too, that the prayer is powerful and effective. I have been so blessed to see God answering my prayers, even though they are not always answered the way I would like them to be. Sometimes God says to wait on Him, and other times he says no to some of my prayers, but one thing I do know is that God always answers for my greatest good.

One of my answered prayers is that I hear about the success that so many women are having in their journeys. I pray that your journey has brought you success too, and that you have learned and grown in your own walk with God. Continue walking in prayer and continue to form great habits and you will win the race you are running.

Someday perhaps we'll see with greater clarity how God has answered all of our prayers, and we may also understand more about the ways in which God works through our prayers. Until that day, remember that your prayers are powerful and effective, and through prayer you can move mountains. He is faithful and God does answer our prayers.

Extra Reading

"Is anyone among you in trouble? Let them pray. Is anyone happy? Let them sing songs of praise. Is anyone among you sick? Let them call the elders of the church to pray over them and anoint them with oil in the name of the Lord. And the prayer offered in faith will make the sick person well; the Lord will raise them up. If they have sinned, they will be forgiven. Therefore confess your sins to each other and pray for each other so that you may be healed. The prayer of a righteous person is powerful and effective."

(James 5: 13-16, NIV)

Prayer Journal

Take some time to reflect on what this means to you. Write your thoughts in your prayer journal.

Day 15

"Trust in the Lord with all your heart and lean not on your own understanding in all your ways submit to him, and he will make your paths straight."

(Proverbs 3:5-6, NIV)

Making The Right Decision

The decisions we make every day are based very largely on our own perspectives and our own worldview. Do you find it difficult to make a decision or do you make a quick decision that comes from your gut or your instinct?

You may find that it's relatively easy to identify and resist the big temptations. Therefore, it is painless for you to make these decisions. The truth is that the big issues of life, the major decisions, usually begin with smaller choices. The little decisions often seem harmless enough in the moment, but they can have long lasting effects on your life.

In Matthew 4, the devil challenges Jesus about his identity, power and steadfastness. Twice he says, "If you are the Son of God... "If you're really who you claim to be, then you should be able to turn stones to bread and jump off cliffs."

Jesus makes the right choice; He knows how to resist the devil's attempt to provoke him. He responds, "Away from me, Satan! For it is written, 'Worship the Lord your God, and serve him only'" (NIV). Jesus resisted the devil's temptations by relying on the truth of God's Word.

The Bible declares you can do all things through Christ. You are more than a conqueror! God affirms He will supply all your needs according to His limitless resources. Remember what's true and right. Your body is a temple of the Holy Spirit. This is truth! Therefore, nourish your body with the right choices today. Do not start second-guessing what God has called you to accomplish. If you trust in Him to guide you, He will make your paths straight, as the verse above declares.

Extra Reading

Then Jesus was led by the Spirit into the wilderness to be tempted by the devil. After fasting forty days and forty nights, he was hungry. The tempter came to him and said, "If you are the Son of God, tell these stones to become bread."

Jesus answered, "It is written: 'Man shall not live on bread alone, but on every word that comes from the mouth of God.' Then the devil took him to the holy city and had him stand on the highest point of the temple. "If you are the Son of God," he said, "throw yourself down. For it is written:"'He will command his angels concerning you, and they will lift you up in their hands, so that you will not strike your foot against a stone.'" Jesus answered him, "It is also written: 'Do not put the Lord your God to the test.'" Again, the devil took him to a very high mountain and showed him all the kingdoms of the world and their splendor. "All this I will give you," he said, "if you will bow down and worship me." Jesus said to him, "Away from me, Satan! For it is written: 'Worship the Lord your God, and serve him only.'" Then the devil left him, and angels came and attended him.

(Matthew 4:1-11, NIV)

Jesus resisted the greatest temptations and made the right decisions by relying on the truth of God's word. When we follow Jesus, we can make the right decisions too. We only need to trust in Him and rely on the promises of God.

Prayer Journal

Take some time to reflect on what this means to you. Write your thoughts in your prayer journal.

Day 16

_____

"Can any one of you by worrying add a single hour to your life?"

(Matthew 6:27, NIV)

Life Without Worries

Are you worried about making it through today? Do you have cares right now that are keeping you from enjoying a happy, healthy life?

When worries or fears constantly distract us from the present moment or from being joyful, we become unhealthy, unhappy, unproductive, and unable to hear God. When we constantly live with worry, our minds become tired and so do our bodies. We tire ourselves out being stressed and anxious, and then wonder why we have no energy left for our daily tasks.

On top of that, stress is one of the absolute worst things for our bodies. Stress can harm our bodies and actually cause us to gain weight. Stress leaves us vulnerable to illness, which only increases worry and reinforces the vicious cycle.

When we worry, we also miss out on hearing from God. We may cry out for his guidance, but if we are not listening to His voice, our minds become clouded and we can't see what's right in front of us. Jesus said in Matthew 6:27 "Can any one of you by worrying add a single hour to your life?" (NIV) The answer is clearly no.

Jesus goes on to tell us that God looks after the flowers and the grass in the field with great care, but the care He gives to those who love Him is wonderful and marvellous. That's a huge WOW.

Being at peace makes us open to what God wants to reveal to us today. I remember worrying about my husband as he worked on all the major highways by himself as a law enforcement officer. I realized very early on in our married life that If I didn't stay in the present moment and continue to give my worries to God, my anxious thoughts would take me down a path of fear and dread. I had to decide to trust Jesus, and then decide to release my worries to God each day and trust him enough to take care of my husband, which He always did.

It sounds easy enough, but in all honesty, it's not always easy to give our worries over to God. We seem to surrender them to Jesus, but we grab hold of them again all too quickly. So how do we give our cares and worries over to God and leave them with him?

The solution to our worries is to seek first the kingdom of God and all his righteousness. "Do not worry about tomorrow for tomorrow will worry about itself, for each day has enough trouble of its own." (Matthew 6:34, NIV)

Then the peace that surpasses all understanding will cover us and we can focus on what we need to do…to seek first the kingdom of God.

We need to take one day at a time, and sometimes it is one hour at a time or even one minute at a time. Think about being in the present moment right now and recite the scripture above. We know that the Bible tells us to cast all our cares upon Him for he cares for us. God loves us more than we love each other, and He wants the very best for our lives. We can surrender our fears and worries to Him and leave them there. Each day we surrender to God, and let go of the outcome. Each day we give him our worries and each day God is in control. You can do this today with God's help. God cares about your body. He cares about your health and your journey. He cares about you, so give your worries to Him and start feeling the peace that surpasses all understanding today.

""Therefore I tell you, do not worry about your life, what you will eat or drink; or about your body, what you will wear. Is not life more than food, and the body more than clothes? Look at the birds of the air; they do not sow or reap or store away in barns, and yet your heavenly Father feeds them. Are you not much more valuable than they? Can any one of you by worrying add a single hour to your life?

Extra Reading

"And why do you worry about clothes? See how the flowers of the field grow. They do not labor or spin. Yet I tell you that not even Solomon in all his splendor was dressed like one of these. If that is how God clothes the grass of the field, which is here today and tomorrow is thrown into the fire, will he not much more clothe you—you of little faith? So do not worry, saying, 'What shall we eat?' or 'What shall we drink?' or 'What shall we wear?' For the pagans run after all these things, and your heavenly Father knows that you need them. But seek first his kingdom and his righteousness, and all these things will be given to you as well. Therefore do not worry about tomorrow, for tomorrow will worry about itself. Each day has enough trouble of its own."

(Matthew 6: 25-34, NIV)

Prayer Journal

Take some time to reflect on what this means to you. Write your thoughts in your prayer journal.

Day 17

"Let us come before him with thanksgiving and extol him with music and song."

(Psalm 95:2, NIV)

Celebration

It may seem strange to you to talk about celebration; however, I believe God wants us to celebrate with Him each day. Our faith in God and knowing what Christ did for us on the cross should cause us to celebrate each day. He died to give us life, and to have life abundant!

Sometimes we forget to stop and celebrate the small things, to smell the roses, to look at a butterfly and marvel, to understand that our Creator wants us to celebrate life.

Jesus also celebrated life. He attended weddings where He turned water into wine. Jesus raised the dead - a celebration indeed! We find plenty of examples of celebrating in the Bible.

One example is when King David was dancing in the streets. Another celebration is found in the book of Esther when Esther played a huge role in saving her people. God wants us to rejoice, to be glad and shout for joy.

One of my favourite stories in the Bible is the story about the celebration of the prodigal son in Luke 15:20-32. "So he got up and went to his father. But while he was still a long way off, his father saw him and was filled with compassion for him; he ran to his son, threw his arms around him and kissed him. The son said to him, 'Father, I have sinned against heaven and against you. I am no longer worthy to be called your son.' But the father said to his servants, 'Quick! Bring the best robe and put it on him. Put a ring on his finger and sandals on his feet. Bring the fattened calf and kill it. Let's have a feast and celebrate. For this son of mine was dead and is alive again; he was lost and is found.' So they began to Celebrate!" (NIV).

A wayward son came home and this was a cause for a cele-bration. As you think about this, what are some of the things you can celebrate today? Maybe you can celebrate the joy your family brings you, or the joy your church family is to you. Maybe you are celebrating reaching your goals, or maybe you are celebrating the fact that your weight loss journey is going well. Each day should cause us to celebrate.

Celebration is a very important part of our life, and we should make it a priority each day. I am celebrating that you are here reading this with me today!

Extra Reading

"Jesus continued: "There was a man who had two sons. The younger one said to his father, 'Father, give me my share of the estate.' So he divided his property between them.

"Not long after that, the younger son got together all he had, set off for a distant country and there squandered his wealth in wild living. After he had spent everything, there was a severe famine in that whole country, and he began to be in need. So he went and hired himself out to a citizen of that country, who sent him to his fields to feed pigs. He longed to fill his stomach with the pods that the pigs were eating, but no one gave him anything.

"When he came to his senses, he said, 'How many of my father's hired servants have food to spare, and here I am starving to death! I will set out and go back to my father and say to him: Father, I have sinned against heaven and against you. I am no longer worthy to be called your son; make me like one of your hired servants.' So he got up and went to his father.

"But while he was still a long way off, his father saw him and was filled with compassion for him; he ran to his son, threw his arms around him and kissed him.

"The son said to him, 'Father, I have sinned against heaven and against you. I am no longer worthy to be called your son.'

"But the father said to his servants, 'Quick! Bring the best robe and put it on him. Put a ring on his finger and sandals on his feet. Bring the fattened calf and kill it. Let's have a feast and celebrate. For this son of mine was dead and is alive again; he was lost and is found.' So they began to celebrate.

"Meanwhile, the older son was in the field. When he came near the house, he heard music and dancing. So he called one of the servants and asked him what was going on. 'Your brother has come,' he replied, 'and your father has killed the fattened calf because he has him back safe and sound.'

"The older brother became angry and refused to go in. So his father went out and pleaded with him. But he answered his father, 'Look! All these years I've been slaving for you and never disobeyed your orders. Yet you never gave me even a young goat so I could celebrate with my friends. But when this son of yours who has squandered your property with prostitutes comes home, you kill the fattened calf for him!'

"'My son,' the father said, 'you are always with me, and everything I have is yours. But we had to celebrate and be glad, because this brother of yours was dead and is alive again; he was lost and is found.'"

(Luke 15:11-32, NIV)

⸺

Prayer Journal

Take some time to reflect on what this means to you. Write your thoughts in your prayer journal.

Day 18

"Love one another, even as I have loved you."

(John 13:34, NIV)

Caring For One Another

Are you ever surprised by people and how they treat each other? Do you ever ask yourself what makes someone really caring and another person harsh and insensitive when both have grown up in the same environment or family? It's puzzling, right?

An interesting book from a psychologist who was sent into a concentration camp in Germany marveled at the fact that while some people turned into selfish, bloodthirsty people, others turned into caring, compassionate individuals who were almost saintly.

The world can be very harsh. Friends can be harsh, and even your family members can be harsh. Sometimes forgiving these people and moving on from their harsh words is easier said than done. I remember a time when I was in elementary school when someone told me I was fat. It was a very cutting remark which had a big effect on me for many years. It was a great struggle for me in my teen years to cope with this limiting belief that replayed over and over in my mind. On my graduation day, all dressed up in my gown with my hair done and looking gorgeous, my Dad told me how beautiful I was. This was the beginning of my turnaround, my transformation from this very hurtful, uncaring remark. Words can really hurt and bruise us, but in the midst of these troubles, God still calls us to forgive and care for others, even to those who have wronged us.

The real question is: How do we care for one another? My father didn't even know how much his caring words meant to me way back then and still today. Those words changed my life!

You might never know how your words will affect someone else in a positive or a negative way. So be sure to care for one another with positive words that are not hurtful. We need to look to the Bible. Just before he faced the cross, Jesus gave his disciples a new commandment: "…love one another, even as I have loved you…" (John 13:34, NIV). Loving one another is one of the greatest keys. Jesus cares for you and I each day. He says we don't need to worry about tomorrow, because He looks after the sparrows, and how much more does he care for us?

Let's lift each other up and care for one another in love. Reach out today and tell someone you care for them. You just never know how your words could change their life...and yours!

Extra Reading

"Jesus entered Jericho and was passing through. A man was there by the name of Zacchaeus; he was a chief tax collector and was wealthy. He wanted to see who Jesus was, but because he was short he could not see over the crowd. So he ran ahead and climbed a sycamore-fig tree to see him, since Jesus was coming that way.

When Jesus reached the spot, he looked up and said to him, "Zacchaeus, come down immediately. I must stay at your house today." So he came down at once and welcomed him gladly.

All the people saw this and began to mutter, "He has gone to be the guest of a sinner."

But Zacchaeus stood up and said to the Lord, "Look, Lord! Here and now I give half of my possessions to the poor, and if I have cheated anybody out of anything, I will pay back four times the amount."

Jesus said to him, "Today salvation has come to this house, because this man, too, is a son of Abraham. For the Son of Man came to seek and to save the lost.""

(Luke 19:1-10, NIV)

The words Jesus spoke to Zacchaeus that day changed his life forever. Let's learn to follow Jesus' example and care for people so that we too will have an impact on the lives of others.

Prayer Journal

Take some time to reflect on what this means to you. Write your thoughts in your prayer journal.

Day 19

"Love the Lord your God with all your heart and with all your soul and with all your mind and with all your strength. The second is this: 'Love your neighbor as yourself. there is no other commandment greater than these.'"

(Mark 12:30-31, NIV)

Love Your Neighbour

Have you ever been asked for money from someone on the street? I'm sure you have had this experience; I would say we all have, but I am often curious as to why the person needs money. Are they hungry? Do they want to buy clothes? Do they want to buy medication for their family? Do they want to support their addiction?

One time when I was asked for money, I asked the person if they were hungry. This particular person pointed to his stomach and said he was very hungry. I somehow wasn't convinced, but when I invited him to the nearest grocery store to buy him some groceries, to my surprise he agreed to come. He was hungry so I fed him.

I believe helping your neighbour in this way is "loving your neighbour." In both the Old and New Testaments we are commanded to love our neighbors as ourselves. What does this mean to you?

On several occasions Jesus himself says this is a part of fulfilling God's law. Again and again he shows us how to love others. Firstly he says, "Love the Lord your God with all your heart and with all your soul and with all your mind and with all your strength." The second is this: "Love your neighbor as yourself. There is no commandment greater than these." (Mark 12:30–31, NIV).

I want to live my life loving my neighbour and not being suspicious or judgemental. If God calls me to love the street person, I want to listen and love my neighbor the way Jesus would.

Certainly there are people who might try to take advantage of us, but that doesn't excuse us from helping those who are in real need. Let's not allow our suspicions and cynical attitudes to stop us from showing God's love to our neighbors and from fulfilling God's commandment to us.

Who do you see as your neighbour? Your neighbour might quite literally be your next door neighbour or it could be the person beside you in the grocery store, or maybe it is the panhandler on the street or possibly your friend from another city. What can you do to love your neighbour today?

Extra Reading

"One of the teachers of the law came and heard them debating. Noticing that Jesus had given them a good answer, he asked him, "Of all the commandments, which is the most important?"

"The most important one," answered Jesus, "is this: 'Hear, O Israel: The Lord our God, the Lord is one. Love the Lord your God with all your heart and with all your soul and with all your mind and with all your strength.' The second is this: 'Love your neighbor as yourself.' There is no commandment greater than these."

"Well said, teacher," the man replied. "You are right in saying that God is one and there is no other but him. To love him with all your heart, with all your understanding and with all your strength, and to love your neighbor as yourself is more important than all burnt offerings and sacrifices.""

(Mark 12:28-33, NIV)

Which neighbour will you love today?

Prayer Journal

Take some time to reflect on what this means to you. Write your thoughts in your prayer journal.

Day 20

"Give careful thought to the paths for your feet and be steadfast in all your ways."

(Proverbs 4:26, NIV)

Square Peg In A Round Hole

Have you ever tried to put a square peg into a round hole? It really doesn't work!

Maybe you feel like a square peg in a round hole because you have tried to fit into a mold that just isn't you. Maybe you have strived to become a musician, but you just don't have the beat. Maybe you are an accountant by trade, but your heart says you're a teacher, so you just don't fit the mark.

Maybe you have tried all the yo-yo diets out there and they just haven't worked for you. You may have felt that you were pushing and straining to get that square peg into the right hole or the right weight loss plan, but so far it still hasn't worked for you. In fact, nothing has worked for you. The peg doesn't match the hole.

If this is the case for you with weight loss, so many of the diet plans out there don't work because they are not the right plan for your body. The peg doesn't fit for a reason! Has this left you feeling defeated? Using the wrong plan with the wrong coach will keep you getting the same negative results over and over. I have heard this called the definition of insanity, doing the same thing over and over and expecting a different result.

Well, it's time to feel like you are hitting the mark! It's time to find the right hole, either a round peg in a round hole or a square peg in a square hole. God wants to be at the center of our life in every aspect of our lives, whether it's with the job we are working at or with the nutrition plan we are on. God calls us to give careful thought to our paths, and invite him into every situation, even our weight loss plan.

When God's at the center, it flows and it works. Proverbs 4:26 says "Give careful thought to the paths for your feet and be steadfast in all your ways" (NIV). Lay it before God and let Him open the doors. If He is in it, it's remarkable how you will fit! You will grow and learn and your interest and commitment to living a happy, healthy life will percolate, just like a coffee pot.

When God is invited into your journey, he will help you fit into the right mold. In fact, God will mold you until you are the vessel he wants you to be, whether it's round or square. Just like the coffee pot percolates, so too will God continue to chip and sculpt away at our outer shells, molding us so that we fit into the right peg. God knows the path we need to take, we just need to be willing to step onto the right path.

———

Extra Reading

"God has no limitations in His ability to perform miracles; nothing is impossible. I am really fond of this scripture from 1 Thessalonians 5:23. "May God himself, the God of peace, sanctify you through and through. May your whole spirit, soul and body be kept blameless at the coming of our Lord Jesus Christ. The one who calls you is faithful, and he will do it" (NIV).

Yes, the one who calls you is faithful, and if you follow His leading and direction, You will have success. You are the right peg and God is shaping you into the woman he is calling you to be. You will be the right peg in the right hole.

———

Prayer Journal

Take some time to reflect on what this means to you. Write your thoughts in your prayer journal.

Day 21

"Ask, and it will be given to you; seek, and you will find; knock, and it will be opened to you. For everyone who asks receives, and he who seeks finds, and to him who knocks it will be opened."

(Matthew 7:7-8, NIV)

Knock And The Door Will Be Opened To You

Have you ever heard of a secret prayer?

Some people use Matthew 7 as their secret prayer. The reason they call this a secret is because in this verse there are three main components or commands, each with a promise that God calls us to do. The secret is that you need to do all 3, not just 1or 2. Let's take a look at this powerful and profound revelation.

Jesus himself says: ""Ask, and it will be given to you; seek, and you will find; knock, and it will be opened to you. For everyone who asks receives, and he who seeks finds, and to him who knocks it will be opened. If you then, being evil, know how to give good gifts to your children, how much more will your Father who is in heaven give good things to those who ask Him!" (Matthew 7:7-8, NIV) Wow - isn't that powerful? Jesus doesn't say it might happen....He says "it will!" That is so powerful.

If we ask in accordance with His will, we will receive, we will find, and the door will be opened. There are three promises, but there are three things to do! So often we might ask, but we don't seek. We might seek, but we don't open the door. We might knock, but we don't ask! Get the picture? The secret is in doing all three. God wants us to take action. He wants us to ask, seek and knock.

This is a very good thought for all of us on this journey to a happier, healthier lifestyle. When we pray we need to ask the Lord to help guide us each day in our weight loss journey, in loving ourselves and in our commitment to see it through to the end to reach our goals and then, of course, to maintain this goal. It will be given to you, for everyone who asks will receive. God wants you to live a healthy life, so this is in accordance with His will.

When we seek, we will continue to find each step that is required to create a new lifestyle with better eating habits every day so our success continues. The verse says that those who seek will find. You will find strength each day.

And finally, if you continue to knock everyday and follow His steps, the door of success will be opened to you. You will be living a happy, healthy life each day with His guidance and in His will.

I know that I have simplified this verse to fit this scenario, but I do believe that God's plan is for you and I to live a life through the secrets of doing these three things: Ask, Seek and Knock!

I'm so thankful that you are taking the steps necessary to living your best life on purpose. I do believe in this secret prayer with all my heart and my prayer for you today is that you Ask God to guide you each day of your life. I pray that you continue to seek His guidance everyday, and I pray that you keep knocking so that God will open the door for you to keep following in His footsteps.

When we are living in the will of Our Father, who is in heaven, He wants to give good things to those who ask Him!

———

Extra Reading

""Ask and it will be given to you; seek and you will find; knock and the door will be opened to you. For everyone who asks receives; the one who seeks finds; and to the one who knocks, the door will be opened.

"Which of you, if your son asks for bread, will give him a stone? Or if he asks for a fish, will give him a snake? If you, then, though you are evil, know how to give good gifts to your children, how much more will your Father in heaven give good gifts to those who ask him! So in everything, do to others what you would have them do to you, for this sums up the Law and the Prophets."

(Matthew 7:7-11, NIV)

———

Prayer Journal

Take some time to reflect on what this means to you. Write your thoughts in your prayer journal.

Day 22

"Lord, the God of heaven, the great and awesome God, who keeps his covenant of love with those who love him and keep his commandments, let your ear be attentive and your eyes open to hear the prayer your servant is praying before you day and night for your servants, the people of Israel."

(Nehemiah 1:5, NIV)

Being A Leader

When you think of "leading from the front," what comes into your mind?

"Leading from the front," means being visible and engaging at the front while still being able to see the forest through the trees. This saying actually comes from a concourse of houses that were designed by the architect John Wood. There was a tree planted directly in front of these houses, and it grew quite large. So people began to exclaim: "You can't see the Wood for the tree!"

I believe this is the type of leader who sees what's going on both up front and at the rear; it is a leader who can help direct those who don't see all the angles. They understand the bigger picture and can help bring the team together so that all the work gets done and in a timely fashion.

Leaders who have this style use the words "Follow me!" Great leaders in the Bible were great prayer warriors as well, which is the reason they had the strength and ability to lead from the front. There are many Bible stories of people leading from the front.

One of my favorite stories is in the book of Nehemiah. Nehemiah was a Jewish biblical figure who appeared in the historical events in Israel during the Jewish Exile. Nehemiah was a cupbearer in the king's palace (King Artaxerxes of Persia). Today we would think of him as more like a house manager who managed the king's palace. He was distinguished, efficient, and noble...and the king loved him. He knew all the angles of the palace.

Nehemiah was also known as a man who feared God; people knew he was a godly man. There is a connection here, because of Nehemia's great faith and as a man of prayer, he was able to lead from the front, even while being in exile. God gave him wisdom and power and he could see the woods through the trees.

The journey that you may have embarked on to live a happy, healthy life can be similar to leading from the front. If you are a mother or a grandmother, then you will be leading from the front in your kitchen. You are probably preparing most of the meals for your family so you are therefore leading the way in eating healthy or unhealthy. You know what each person likes and dislikes and you have input into what nutrients go into their bodies. You may also be leading your extended family or friends as you show them how you are changing your daily eating habits. In this healthy lifestyle journey that you have embarked upon, you have the opportunity to share and encourage others along the way as well, which is still another way of leading from the front.

God calls us to lead in different ways and in different capacities at different stages of our lives, so how are you leading in your life today? Maybe it's through your role as a mother or grandmother, or maybe it's through the role of being a good friend. However you are being used, just remember that we can all learn lessons from the Bible from others that have gone on before us that will help to stretch and push us out of our comfort level in order to be good leaders.

I hope I have inspired you in some little way to step out and lead which will inspire others to also live a happy, healthy life.

Extra Reading

"The words of Nehemiah son of Hakaliah:

In the month of Kislev in the twentieth year, while I was in the citadel of Susa, Hanani, one of my brothers, came from Judah with some other men, and I questioned them about the Jewish remnant that had survived the exile, and also about Jerusalem.

They said to me, "Those who survived the exile and are back in the province are in great trouble and disgrace. The wall of Jerusalem is broken down, and its gates have been burned with fire."

When I heard these things, I sat down and wept. For some days I mourned and fasted and prayed before the God of heaven. Then I said:

"Lord, the God of heaven, the great and awesome God, who keeps his covenant of love with those who love him and keep his commandments, let your ear be attentive and your eyes open to hear the prayer your servant is praying before you day and night for your servants, the people of Israel. I confess the sins we Israelites, including myself and my father's family, have committed against you. We have acted very wickedly toward you. We have not obeyed the commands, decrees and laws you gave your servant Moses.

"Remember the instruction you gave your servant Moses, saying, 'If you are unfaithful, I will scatter you among the nations, but if you return to me and obey my commands, then even if your exiled people are at the farthest horizon, I will gather them from there and bring them to the place I have chosen as a dwelling for my Name.'

"They are your servants and your people, whom you redeemed by your great strength and your mighty hand. Lord, let your ear be attentive to the prayer of this your servant and to the prayer of your servants who delight in revering your name. Give your servant success today by granting him favor in the presence of this man."

I was cupbearer to the king."

(Nehemiah 1, NIV)

Prayer Journal

Take some time to reflect on what this means to you. Write your thoughts in your prayer journal.

Day 23

"Do not neglect to show hospitality to strangers, for by this some have entertained angels without knowing it."

(Hebrews 13:2, NIV)

Entertaining Angels

The word hospitality can feel very overwhelming at times because to some people this means creating a 5-course meal that is fit for a king. It means working in the kitchen creating elaborate, gourmet meals with lavish preparations. We may feel we just can't "keep up."

However, the Bible offers a very different idea of hospitality. Biblical hospitality does not necessarily mean welcoming people into a well-groomed home with a 5-star gourmet meal. It may involve feeding the poor, bringing someone a home-cooked meal, or simply welcoming strangers into your home or community and serving them a cup of tea. What happened to the days of simply serving a steaming bowl of hot soup?

It may seem daunting, but the Bible is pretty clear that we should be entertaining angels! Hebrews 13:2 says, "Do not neglect to show hospitality to strangers, for by this some have entertained angels without knowing it." Wow! Just imagine... you could have angels in your midst without even knowing it. This can be scary and exciting all at the same time. Have you ever considered hosting strangers?

In today's world, we have become fearful of strangers; we don't talk to strangers anymore, let alone consider hosting strangers in our house. What does hospitality mean to you? When was the last time someone was hospitable to you? And when was the last time you were hospitable to someone else?

Think about how you can show hospitality in your life today. If a stranger or a needy friend appeared at your door, what would you do? I believe you can even show hospitality inside different internet groups, like on Facebook. Maybe caring and reaching out to someone who needs a boost of encouragement is another form of hospitality or a way of "entertaining angels unaware."

I know that in my own life I have reached out to a few strangers at different times and I have been the one who received the biggest blessing, even as I sought to bless them. It is through serving others that we feel a sense of fulfillment and happiness whether we are entertaining angels or just serving to please our Lord.

You never know how your words will touch someone's life. Use your God-given wisdom, and if God asks you to open your door to a lonely neighbor or a lonely internet friend, what a wonderful opportunity for you to show hospitality. Ask God to show you how you can be hospitable today and

God will bless you for reaching out. You never know just when you will be entertaining angels.

———

Extra Reading

"Keep on loving one another as brothers and sisters. Do not forget to show hospitality to strangers, for by so doing some people have shown hospitality to angels without knowing it. Continue to remember those in prison as if you were together with them in prison, and those who are mistreated as if you yourselves were suffering."

Hebrews 13:1-3, NIV)

———

Prayer Journal

Take some time to reflect on what this means to you. Write your thoughts in your prayer journal.

Day 24

"Come to me, all you who are weary and burdened, and I will give you rest."

(Matthew 11:28, NIV)

Bearing One Another's Burdens

Have you ever been in need? Has anyone ever helped you bear one of your burdens? If so, you may have seen how God worked in your life by having someone come alongside you who helped to lift you up and bear your burden with you.

It is very comforting to know that God watches over us when we need someone to help carry us through a difficult time. Sometimes God places people in our lives at certain times who are in need. God is aware of what they lack, and He has given you the resources or the ability to meet those needs.

God does nothing by accident. God may be placing someone with a need in front of you because He knows you have the ability to help bear that particular burden; you are chosen by God to help meet that need. God wants to use you in these situations to bring glory and honor to Him. Bearing one another's burdens can feel overwhelming at times. However, recognizing a need in someone's life can be one of the greatest invitations from God we will ever experience.

Rather than looking at each new burden as one more drain on our time, energy, or finances, let's learn to thank God that he has blessed us with the resources to lighten someone's load. Galatians 6:2 says, "Bear one another's burdens and so fulfill the law of Christ" (NIV). It is our duty as fellow believers to help bear one another's burdens. When others have burdens too heavy to bear, they stagger, and we can help steady the load. If their burdens become overwhelming, they may stumble, and it is our duty to help lift them up. Helping fellow believers carry the weight of their burdens is one of the practical ways in which we should practice. Ask God to help you with bearing one another's burdens, so that you are fulfilling the law of Christ.

Maybe you have been burdened and overwhelmed with struggling to lose weight. This might be a burden you bear and you may feel you need someone to help carry you through the next day of this journey. Or on the flip side, maybe you know someone who has this burden and you're the one to help lift and encourage them back up.

We as believers are asked to bring our cares and our burdens to God. Jesus tells us to come to Him and He will give us rest. Let's be sure to trust our Savior enough to give us the rest we need for today.

If you are weary today, Jesus is there waiting for you.

Extra Reading

"Brothers and sisters, if someone is caught in a sin, you who live by the Spirit should restore that person gently. But watch yourselves, or you also may be tempted. Carry each other's burdens, and in this way you will fulfill the law of Christ."

(Galatians 6:1-2, NIV)

Prayer Journal

Take some time to reflect on what this means to you. Write your thoughts in your prayer journal.

Day 25

"Come away by yourselves to a secluded place and rest a while."

(Mark 6:31, NIV)

Taking A Rest

Proper rest seems to be a lost art in our modern culture. It sure feels like we've exchanged old-fashioned value for a hectic, fast-paced, breakneck speed of life. The busier we get, the more our fervor and passion disintegrate, while our blood pressure elevates. We pack too much into each 24-hour time span and this is unsustainable! Then on top of our own chaotic schedules, there are the demands from others that are deemed urgent enough to be placed upon us and we quickly forget or have no time to take care of ourselves.

Rest is one of the first things we give up, which is the most necessary component for living a happy, healthy life. Rest is part of the balance, and so often we neglect this single action from our lifestyle.

When Jesus sent His disciples off on a ministry assignment (Mark 6:7-11), He didn't shield them from the fact that their journey would not be easy. So as their first order of business upon returning, Jesus greeted them with clear instructions to rest: "He said to them, 'Come away by yourselves to a secluded place and rest a while'" (Mark6:31a, NIV). It wasn't a friendly suggestion. It was a clear instruction from Jesus. It was like Jesus saying… "Here's what you're going to do now. You've been through a lot, and there is so much more that remains to be done, so for now, come and rest and take a break by yourselves."

One of the things I am passionate about is helping women learn to take care of themselves. So often women put themselves last, or never really take a break. Women tend to feel guilty for giving themselves a bit of a rest.

I believe it's time to stop feeling guilty or selfish for taking time for yourself; you must take care of yourself so that you can continue to care for those you love. Women, in particular, seem to neglect taking a rest because there is always another task waiting to get done. It is important to have that balance and to look after your body, so that you can be the Woman Chosen For Greatness that God destined you to be.

Here are a few questions to ask yourself.

- Do you feel guilty for taking time away to regroup and recharge?
- Do you feel guilty for saying no?
- Do you feel like you're wasting time if every space on your calendar is not filled up?

- Do you feel selfish if you take a rest from your to-do list?

Quiet time is not an excuse for the lazy, but a wise investment for the diligent. It's for those who are committed to being active servants and followers of Jesus Christ instead of slaves to the tyranny of urgent busyness and activity.

By prioritizing rest for ourselves and those we love, we might just rediscover the joy we thought had been lost forever. Rest is the time when your inner cells heal and repair, so please take care of yourself and take time for rest.

Extra Reading

"Then, because so many people were coming and going that they did not even have a chance to eat, he said to them, "Come with me by yourselves to a quiet place and get some rest.""

(Mark 6:31, NIV)

Prayer Journal

Take some time to reflect on what this means to you. Write your thoughts in your prayer journal.

Day 26

"Gray hair is a crown of splendor; it is attained in the way of righteousness."

(Proverbs 16:31, NIV)

Aging Well

Are you aging gracefully?

Age is just a number, just like the number on the scale. You might not like the numbers, but they do not define us nor are we bound by that number. As we learn and grow through life, we have different experiences that mold us into the beautiful woman God wants us to be. With every season in life, we have a life to live, not to hide.

Society, the media and magazines suggest that we should never grow old. Here is what a wrinkle-free woman says, "I intend to fight it every step of the way!" Our culture seems to tell us that we shouldn't have wrinkles or gray hair, but that is not how God designed our bodies to stay. Our bodies change with every season of life and with God's help we must learn to adapt.

So what does God say about it all? If we listen to the One Who created us, we will hear all about grace and goodness; not fear and resistance. Proverbs 16:31 says: "Gray hair is a crown of splendor; it is attained in the way of right-eousness" (NIV).

The more years we live, the more experiences we are given to learn from, and the more wisdom and perspective we gain to see life in new and beautiful ways. It's not always easy for women to see themselves getting older or adding another wrinkle to their face, but we can learn to grow old gracefully with the promises of God's word. He cares for us always.

In Titus 2:3-5, Paul reminds the older women of their great purpose – by living reverent lives of love, self-control, purity and kindness, they will bless and nurture the hearts of the younger women and their families. The generations to come depend on the willingness of the older women to share what God has done for them.

God wants older women to teach the younger women and to care for those coming behind them.

We are all Women Chosen For Greatness, and we want to leave our legacy with the next generation. This is a true blessing.

Aging can be seen as a loss of control, but really it's a blessing from God. Maybe your body is not able to do what it once could, maybe your memory is not as sharp, maybe you need more help than you used to, but the truth is, you have never been in control anyway! From the moment you were created - whether you realize it or not -

God has always been in control. Aging is just part of God's design.

What you can control in this life is how you treat your body at every age. You can control what you put into it, with regards to food and drink, and you can control how you talk to yourself, with regards to your thoughts.

The way you speak to yourself really does matter. Your words can help you overcome the doubts you have and your words can help you stay focused on what really matters to you. Your words can make you feel better as you age gracefully and strive to live a happier, healthier life.

How can we lean into God as we age, trusting that every day matters, from our first to our last?

Claim His promises today. Sit down with a journal and your Bible and interview yourself about growing older. Here are a few questions to ponder:

Am I afraid of aging? And if so, why?

Once you've recorded your thoughts, find specific promises in God's Word that will help bring you peace and assurance.

Next, choose to make healthy choices. While the human body is not intended to live forever, we can still honor our Creator by making choices that bring us health and strength each day. We are here at this time for a reason – let's not miss the opportunities to help guide and encourage those around us!

Extra Reading

"Gracious words are a honeycomb, sweet to the soul and healing to the bones."

(Proverbs 16:24, NIV)

———

Prayer Journal

Take some time to reflect on what this means to you. Write your thoughts in your prayer journal.

Day 27

"For where your treasure is, there your heart will be also."

(Luke 12:34, NIV)

Finding Your Treasure

What is your most valuable treasure? Is it your family, your grandkids, your possessions, your money, your time? And where do you spend your time?

Think about this: Whatever dominates your conversation is what you treasure, and what you are known for with others is also a good indication of what your treasure is. Jesus said in Luke 12:34 "For where your treasure is, there your heart will be also" (NIV). If you are unsure of where your treasure is, examine where your thoughts are, where your time goes, and where your money is spent.

Many people are quick to claim that God is their first priority, and they fully intend that to be true. Yet their actions often reveal that their treasure is not in God nor

His kingdom, but instead their treasures are the things of this world.

Some people find it difficult to discuss their relationship with God, but they can chatter easily about their family, friends, or hobbies. Some people find it impossible to rise early in order to spend time with God, but they willingly get up at dawn to pursue a hobby. Others find it difficult to give an offering to God, but readily spend lavishly on recreation. And some people boldly approach strangers to sell a product, yet they are painfully timid in telling others about their Savior.

Do you struggle with any of these issues in your life? If you do, please know that you are not alone. I know that I certainly struggle with some of these issues at times. I want my real treasure to be centered on God and his Kingdom, and yet I often find myself falling short. There are so many good treasures, and God does not deny us pleasures, but our real treasure is found in following the will of God and then our lives are greatly fulfilled.

I truly believe that you are a Woman Chosen For Greatness and I know God treasures you beyond your imagination. As you reflect on God's word today, figure out what you really treasure because that is where your heart is also.

You may want to ask your friends what they believe to be your most important treasure. Or ask your children to list the things they see most valuable to you. It may surprise you to know what others consider to be your greatest treasure. This may be a great insight into what your treasure actually is.

Extra Reading

"Someone in the crowd said to him, "Teacher, tell my brother to divide the inheritance with me." Jesus replied, "Man, who appointed me a judge or an arbiter between you?" Then he said to them, "Watch out! Be on your guard against all kinds of greed; life does not consist in an abundance of possessions."

And he told them this parable: "The ground of a certain rich man yielded an abundant harvest. He thought to himself, 'What shall I do? I have no place to store my crops.' "Then he said, 'This is what I'll do. I will tear down my barns and build bigger ones, and there I will store my surplus grain. And I'll say to myself, "You have plenty of grain laid up for many years. Take life easy; eat, drink and be merry."'

"But God said to him, 'You fool! This very night your life will be demanded from you. Then who will get what you have prepared for yourself?'

"This is how it will be with whoever stores up things for themselves but is not rich toward God.""

(Luke 12:13-21, NIV)

Prayer Journal

Take some time to reflect on what this means to you. Write your thoughts in your prayer journal.

Day 28

"But do not forget this one thing, dear friends: With the Lord a day is like a thousand years, and a thousand years are like a day."

(2 Peter 3:8, NIV)

Time

God gives us 24 hours—1,440 minutes—each and every day. We get to choose how to use this time; we can use it wisely or we can waste our time. We must remember though that our time does eventually run out. There will come a day when we are called to account for how we have used the time and all the other resources God has given us.

In Luke 19:11-27 Jesus tells this parable. A man of noble birth, who goes on a journey to be appointed king, gives 10 of his servants ten minas (about three months wages). He tells them to put the money to work. Several servants do this and they get a return on their money. One servant, though, laid his minas away and did nothing, stating that his boss was a hard man and he was afraid. This can be synonymous with time: we can invest our time wisely and get some return on it, or we can waste it away because we are afraid to take action.

God has given each of us spiritual gifts and talents (1Corinthians 12:7-11) and all kinds of other resources. He wants us to use them wisely, just like the king wanted the servants to invest the minas wisely.

How should we then live? I understand that I must use the time I have everyday wisely.

I choose to block some time each day to look after my health and well being. I want this for you too, as I believe our bodies are the temple of the Holy Spirit. In order to live our best life and do the things God calls us to do, we must take care of ourselves. God wants you to take care of yourself, to eat healthy, to move your body so that you can continue to do His work.

As women, we must learn to love ourselves, and not be afraid to take action. Let's not hide our gifts (our minas) in the ground any longer. Let's not allow fear to keep us from investing in ourselves or from taking care of our bodies. It's time to step out of our comfort zone and use the gifts God has given us. Our time is short! The time we have to invest for God is now.

Here is my prayer for you today:

"Lord, bless each hour that you have given me today. Help me to make the most of my precious time in this life. I want to spend my time wisely, without hiding my talents away. Forgive me for the times I have spent in fear or need-less endeavors. Help me to treat my body like a temple so that I am healthy and can continue to serve you and your kingdom without fear."

Extra Reading

"While they were listening to this, he went on to tell them a parable, because he was near Jerusalem and the people thought that the kingdom of God was going to appear at once. He said: "A man of noble birth went to a distant country to have himself appointed king and then to return. So he called ten of his servants and gave them ten minas. 'Put this money to work,' he said, 'until I come back.'

"But his subjects hated him and sent a delegation after him to say, 'We don't want this man to be our king.'

"He was made king, however, and returned home. Then he sent for the servants to whom he had given the money, in order to find out what they had gained with it.

"The first one came and said, 'Sir, your mina has earned ten more.'

"'Well done, my good servant!' his master replied. 'Because you have been trustworthy in a very small matter, take charge of ten cities.'

"The second came and said, 'Sir, your mina has earned five more.'

"His master answered, 'You take charge of five cities.'

"Then another servant came and said, 'Sir, here is your mina; I have kept it laid away in a piece of cloth. I was afraid of you, because you are a hard man. You take out what you did not put in and reap what you did not sow.'

"His master replied, 'I will judge you by your own words, you wicked servant! You knew, did you, that I am a hard man, taking out what I did not put in, and reaping what I did not sow? Why then didn't you put my money on deposit, so that when I came back, I could have collected it with interest?'

"Then he said to those standing by, 'Take his mina away from him and give it to the one who has ten minas.'

"'Sir,' they said, 'he already has ten!'

"He replied, 'I tell you that to everyone who has, more will be given, but as for the one who has nothing, even what they have will be taken away."

(Luke 19:11-27, NIV)

Prayer Journal

Take some time to reflect on what this means to you. Write your thoughts in your prayer journal.

Day 29

"Those who work their land will have abundant food, but those who chase fantasies will have their fill of poverty."

(Proverbs 28:19, NIV)

Abundance Versus Poverty

In the beginning, God's plan for us was abundance. Poverty is one of the curses of the broken law that we live under today and yet Jesus endured the curse for us that we might have an abundant life. We can still have an abundant life today because we have been blessed with so many rich promises of God. We see abundance from God's word starting in the first book of the Bible, in Genesis, where we see the abundance of the heavens, the abundance of water, the earth and all it's abundance like the flowers, the grass, the fruit, the leaves on the trees, the animals and the birds, etc. We read that God saw all creation and it was good. The earth was abundant and free. We can look and see

God's beauty all around us and that makes us rich in His abundant love towards us.

In the Bible Jesus says, "It's more blessed to give than to receive." God gave us the ultimate gift, His son, and because of that we can live an abundant and free life.

If we are always receiving and never giving, we are not enjoying the greater blessings that God wants all His people to enjoy. God so wants us to experience His abundance, more than enough for ourselves that we may share with others. There are many ways of giving; we can give financially or give of ourselves, of our time and our resources. Scripture makes it very clear that it is more blessed to give, so let's start a habit of giving.

It's very easy to get distracted from what God really wants for us here. Proverbs tells us quite frankly that if we are willing to work the land we will have abundance. If we chase after fantasies, we will have our fill of poverty. God has called us to work diligently and to give cheerfully from what we have, as it is more blessed to give than to receive.

Let's shift our focus from negative thoughts to positive thoughts. Many times our actions reflect our mindset. When we are grumbling and complaining, the poverty mindset comes out. When we are grateful and thankful, the abundant mindset comes out.

The Bible says He will provide our needs and Christ has redeemed us from the poverty curse. 2 Corinthians 8:9: "For you know the grace of our Lord Jesus Christ, that though he was rich, yet for your sakes, He became poor so that you through his poverty might become rich" (NIV). We no longer need to be slaves to poverty because we are rich in His blessings.

How can we apply this to our daily lives when we want to live a happy, healthy life. Many people today have a mindset of poverty. They don't see the abundance of God's creation. They aren't happy because they don't see the abundance of sand on a seashore, the abundance of waves in the ocean, the abundance of beauty when they stop to really be still.

We need to open our eyes to see the beauty around us. When we open ourselves up to thanksgiving, we stop seeing a small home, but rather see the beauty in having a home to go to. We stop comparing ourselves to others who have more and rather are thankful for what we are blessed with.

Do you have a poverty or an abundant mindset? Maybe today you want to thank God for the fact that you have abundance in your life. You have abundance in being able to purchase healthy foods to nourish your body. You have an abundance of love from the Creator who for our sakes, became poor.

So let's be thankful for our abundance today. Let's see the cup half full instead of half empty. It's such a different perspective, and it can totally change the entire day for you when you see the abundance rather than the poverty.

The Bible says in Philippians 4:6, Do not be anxious about anything, but in every situation, by prayer and petition, with thanksgiving present your requests to God (NIV).

It is with a grateful heart and an abundant mindset that you will succeed on your journey. Start thanking God for the abundance in your life today.

Extra Reading:

"If you fully obey the Lord your God and carefully follow all his commands I give you today, the Lord your God will set you high above all the nations on earth. All these blessings will come on you and accompany you if you obey the Lord your God."

(Deuteronomy 28:1-2, NIV)

Prayer Journal

Take some time to reflect on what this means to you. Write your thoughts in your prayer journal.

Day 30

"You are the salt of the earth."

(Matthew 5:13, NIV)

Salt Of The Earth

I'm sure you have heard this statement: "You are the salt of the earth." What did Jesus mean when He told His followers that they were "the salt of the earth?" (Matthew 5:13, NIV).

In the ancient world, salt had many uses. It was used to preserve food because without salt, meat and fish would quickly spoil. In a similar way, believers who lose their saltiness or are without salt, soon spoil too.

Salt was also used as a fertilizer. Until the mid-1900s, English farmers added salt to their fields to increase the yield. Salt helped their crops to grow. Salty christians are like fertilizer, encouraging other christians to learn and grow in their faith. As well, the saltiness spreads to nonbelievers and helps them taste and see that the Lord is good.

Another known benefit to salt is that it really brings out the richness, the deep flavors of our food. In the same way, salty believers can enjoy and taste life fully, abundantly, as God intended.

One of my goals is to spread a little salt on you and to encourage you in your walk with God. I hope you draw closer to God, and continue to read daily devotionals to keep learning and growing.

I am also motivated to be the salt (encouragement) for you in your healthy lifestyle journey so that you achieve your goals and succeed in living a happy, healthy life the way that God wants you to. I pray that today you will stay focused and keep on track with the goals you set for yourself. Stay salty, keep going, keep learning and growing.

Jesus warned the believers long ago that salt could lose its flavor. Pure salt as we know it, sodium chloride, can't lose its taste. However, in ancient Israel, the farmers would dig for salt from the shores of the Dead Sea. Although it was called salt and looked like salt, it was mixed with other substances as well. Farmers would gather a pile of the salty material to use on their crops, but as soon as the rains came, the pure salt would drain away. What was left looked like salt, and yet it had lost all its saltiness. Let's remain steadfast in God's word so that we do not lose our saltiness like the farmers did. Let's preserve the real pure salt and keep spreading and encouraging others to taste of God's goodness.

Extra Reading:

"You are the salt of the earth. But if the salt loses its saltiness, how can it be made salty again? It is no longer good for anything, except to be thrown out and trampled underfoot.

You are the light of the world. A town built on a hill cannot be hidden. Neither do people light a lamp and put it under a bowl. Instead they put it on its stand, and it gives light to everyone in the house. In the same way, let your light shine before others, that they may see your good deeds and glorify your Father in heaven."

(Matthew 5:13-16, NIV)

Prayer Journal

Take some time to reflect on what this means to you. Write your thoughts in your prayer journal.

Made in the USA
Middletown, DE
05 March 2023

26245452R00061